LOW PROTEIN DIET
FOR KIDNEY DISEASE

**The Optimal Nutrition Guide with Delicious
Recipes to Fight Renal Disease**

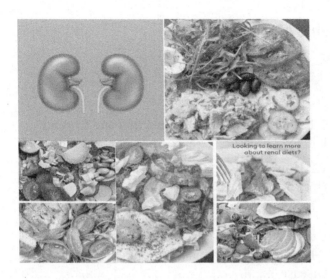

Looking to learn more about renal diets?

Benefits of a low protein diet for kidney health

1. Reduced Kidney Workload
2. Slowed Progression of Kidney Disease
3. Lowered Risk of Proteinuria
4. Better Blood Pressure Control
5. Minimized Risk of Uric Acid Buildup
6. Improved Management of Diabetes
7. Prevention of Malnutrition

Table of Contents

Introduction

In life, we often face unexpected challenges that demand our unwavering strength and resilience. For me, that challenge came in the form of kidney disease, a battle that would forever alter the course of my life. This book, "Low Protein Diet for Kidney Disease," is not just a compilation of recipes and dietary guidelines; it is a testament to my journey of resilience, determination, and triumph over adversity.

Rewind to a few years ago, and I was leading what I believed to be a typical, healthy life. My days were filled with laughter, joy, and seemingly boundless energy. Little did I know that lurking beneath the surface, my kidneys were silently struggling to keep up with the demands of daily life. It wasn't until a routine medical checkup that my world came crashing down. The diagnosis was staggering - chronic kidney disease - an ailment that would forever alter my perception of health and wellness.

The road to recovery was paved with uncertainty, fear, and numerous medical interventions. I found myself grappling with an overwhelming sense of helplessness, unsure of where to turn or what to do. Amidst this chaos, however, I discovered an incredible support system - my family, friends, and the dedicated healthcare professionals who stood by my side, offering unwavering encouragement and guidance.

As I delved deeper into my condition, I became aware of the crucial role diet played in managing kidney disease. Embracing a low protein diet was not an easy feat, but it quickly became my greatest ally in the battle for better kidney health. This dietary change presented challenges, but I approached them with determination, exploring various culinary avenues, and discovering innovative ways to savor flavor without compromising my well-being.

I understand the uncertainty and fear that often accompany a diagnosis of kidney disease, which is why this book is written with compassion and empathy. Whether you are a patient or a caregiver, I hope the practical insights within this book will inspire you to embark on your own transformative path to kidney health.

Together, let us embrace the healing power of nutrition and rewrite our stories of resilience, turning adversity into triumph, and reclaiming the vibrant life that awaits us beyond the confines of kidney disease. Let this book be the beacon that guides you to a brighter, healthier future, one nourishing meal at a time.

Chapter 1: Understanding Kidney Disease and the Role of a Low Protein Diet

1.1 Overview of Kidney Function and Chronic Kidney Disease

These inconspicuous bean-shaped organs buried within our abdominal cavity, the kidneys, serve a critical function in maintaining our body's delicate equilibrium. Their seemingly basic function of filtering waste from the blood and maintaining fluid and electrolyte levels is actually a complicated symphony that orchestrates our overall health. The kidneys operate nonstop, day and night, cleaning our blood and excreting waste items through urine, keeping our systems in balance.

However, life may often throw us unexpected hurdles, and chronic kidney disease (CKD) is one of such challenges for millions of individuals worldwide. Chronic renal disease is a degenerative disorder marked by a persistent reduction in kidney function over time. While it may be asymptomatic at first, CKD can progress quietly, leading to significant consequences including reduced kidney function.

Understanding the complicated dance of kidney function is critical to grasping the significance of properly managing renal illness. As CKD advances, the kidneys become less effective in filtering waste materials, resulting in toxic accumulation in the circulation. Furthermore, weakened kidneys may struggle to maintain the body's fluid balance, leading to edema, high blood pressure, and electrolyte abnormalities.

1.2 How a Low Protein Diet Can Benefit Kidney Health

A glimmer of light appears amid the hardships of chronic renal disease in the shape of a reduced protein diet. As medical research and expertise have progressed, it has become clear that dietary treatments can play an important role in delaying the course of CKD and preserving renal function.

A low protein diet has emerged as a cornerstone in the management of kidney disease, offering a plethora of advantages to people looking to safeguard their kidney function. Reduced protein consumption, particularly from animal sources, puts less burden on the kidneys and allows them to better regulate waste filtration. This decrease in protein consumption reduces the formation of nitrogenous waste, relieving the pressure on the kidneys.

Furthermore, a well-balanced low protein diet can help regulate hypertension and reduce proteinuria, a disease characterized by an excess of protein in the urine. Lowering proteinuria is crucial since it is a sign of kidney injury and, if left untreated, can worsen the deterioration of renal function.

Chapter 2: The Fundamentals of a Low Protein Diet

2.1 Protein Requirements for People with Kidney Disease

Understanding the particular protein requirements of people with renal illness is the first step in demystifying a low protein diet. Protein, the building block of life, is essential for muscular development, tissue repair, and immune system function. Excess protein consumption, on the other hand, might be problematic for persons with impaired renal function.

The kidneys are in charge of filtering waste products from the blood, and protein breakdown produces nitrogenous waste, which the kidneys must discharge via urine. Reduced kidney function in chronic renal disease can obstruct this process, resulting in a buildup of nitrogenous waste in the circulation.

Protein consumption must be tailored to individual needs in order to establish a balance between nutrition and renal function. To establish the ideal protein consumption for your condition, your healthcare team will evaluate your kidney function, general health, and other pertinent aspects. We may prepare the path for a low protein diet that supports kidney function while satisfying our nutritional demands by paying attention to these unique needs.

2.2 Sources of Protein and Their Impact on Kidney Health

The second component of demystifying a low protein diet is to investigate the various protein sources and their influence on kidney function. Not all proteins are created equal, and the origin of protein-rich meals can have a considerable impact on their renal function.

Essential amino acids may be found in animal-based proteins such as meat, poultry, fish, and dairy products. They do, however, have greater levels of phosphorus, a mineral that can build up in the blood and cause issues with renal illness. As a result, people with renal illness may need to limit their consumption of animal-based proteins.

Plant-based proteins, on the other hand, are better for our kidneys. Legumes, lentils, beans, tofu, and other plant-based protein sources are strong in protein but low in phosphorus, making them good alternatives for a low protein diet. By adopting these plant-based alternatives, we not only safeguard our kidneys, but also open the door to a more diversified and enjoyable culinary experience.

2.3 Choosing the Appropriate Protein Amount for Your Condition

The final piece of the puzzle in decoding a low protein diet is calculating the appropriate quantity of protein for your specific condition. This delicate equilibrium requires fine-tuning since it is affected by factors such as renal disease stage, age, weight, and individual dietary demands.

In this process, it is critical to work closely with your healthcare team. Your primary care physician, nephrologist, and registered dietitian will collaborate to develop a specific low protein diet plan that promotes kidney function while delivering adequate nutrition.

As we progress through the chapters, we will discover the skill of creating balanced and delightful low protein meals. We will embrace a reduced protein diet with confidence and conviction now that we have a better grasp of protein requirements, sources, and personalized consumption. Let us begin on this path to greater kidney health together, making every food choice a monument to our dedication to health.

2.4 The Role of a Low Protein Diet in the Management of Kidney Disease

A low protein diet restricts protein consumption, particularly from animal sources, in order to reduce the stress on the kidneys. Individuals with renal illness can maintain an appropriate protein intake while reducing the risk of problems by choosing plant-based proteins that are friendlier on the kidneys.

Adopting a low protein diet demonstrates our dedication to our health and well-being. In the following chapters, we will delve into a treasure mine of delectable low protein recipes and meal planning ideas for making every meal a nutritious and pleasant experience. Let us take ownership of our kidney health together, armed with knowledge of protein's impact and the transformational power of a low protein diet.

Chapter 3: Understanding Kidney Disease

3.1 Blood in Urine (Hematuria)

Hematuria, or blood in the urine, is a frequent symptom that can indicate a variety of renal disorders. Hematuria can be either gross (visible with the naked eye) or microscopic (detectable only with a microscope). In this part, we will look at the many forms of hematuria, their probable causes, and their importance in detecting renal diseases.

3.2 Protein in Urine (Proteinuria)

Proteinuria is defined as the presence of too much protein in the urine. Normally, just a little quantity of protein enters the urine through the kidney filters (glomeruli). Proteinuria occurs when high amounts of protein are lost in the urine as a result of kidney injury or failure. This section will discuss the importance of proteinuria, its probable causes, and its role as an indication of renal disease.

3.3 Kidney Stones (Nephrolithiasis)

Kidney stones are hard mineral and salt deposits that occur in the kidneys and can be painful to move through the urinary canal. This section will provide you an overview of kidney stones, how they occur, risk factors, and various treatments.

Breakfast Recipes

Chia Seed Pudding with Fresh Berries

Ingredients:

2 tablespoons chia seeds

1 cup unsweetened almond milk

1/2 teaspoon vanilla extract

Fresh berries (blueberries, strawberries, raspberries) for topping

Prep Time: 5 minutes (+ 4 hours for chilling)

Instructions:

In a bowl, mix chia seeds, almond milk, and vanilla extract.

Stir well and refrigerate for at least 4 hours or overnight.

Before serving, top with fresh berries.

Oatmeal with Sliced Banana and Cinnamon

Ingredients:

1/2 cup rolled oats

1 cup water or unsweetened almond milk

1 ripe banana, sliced

A pinch of ground cinnamon

Prep Time: 10 minutes

Instructions:

In a saucepan, bring oats and water (or almond milk) to a boil.

Reduce heat and simmer until oats are cooked and creamy.

Top with sliced banana and a sprinkle of cinnamon.

Tofu and Vegetable Scramble

Ingredients:

1/2 cup soft tofu, crumbled

1/4 cup diced bell peppers

1 cup fresh spinach leaves

1/4 cup cherry tomatoes, halved

1/2 teaspoon turmeric powder

Salt and pepper to taste

Prep Time: 15 minutes

Instructions:

In a non-stick skillet, sauté bell peppers until slightly softened.

Add tofu, turmeric, salt, and pepper, and cook for 2 minutes.

Stir in spinach and cherry tomatoes, and cook until wilted.

Quinoa Breakfast Bowl

Ingredients:

1 cup cooked quinoa

2 tablespoons chopped nuts (almonds, walnuts)

2 tablespoons dried cranberries or raisins

1 teaspoon honey or maple syrup

Prep Time: 10 minutes

Instructions:

In a bowl, combine cooked quinoa, nuts, and dried cranberries.

Drizzle with honey or maple syrup and mix well.

Smoothie Bowl with Low Protein Fruits

Ingredients:

1 cup low protein fruits (berries, kiwi, melon)
1/2 cup unsweetened almond milk
1 tablespoon chia seeds
Low protein granola and seeds for topping
Prep Time: 5 minutes

Instructions:

Blend low protein fruits and almond milk until smooth.
Pour the smoothie into a bowl and top with chia seeds, granola, and seeds.

Avocado Toast with Tomato and Basil

Ingredients:

1 ripe avocado, mashed
2 slices of whole-grain bread, toasted
1 medium tomato, sliced
Fresh basil leaves for topping
Prep Time: 5 minutes

Instructions:

Spread mashed avocado evenly on toasted bread slices.

Top with tomato slices and fresh basil leaves.

Blueberry and Almond Muffins

Ingredients:

1 cup almond flour

1/2 cup low protein flour (rice or oat flour)

1/4 cup honey or maple syrup

1/2 teaspoon baking powder

1/2 cup unsweetened almond milk

1/2 cup fresh blueberries

Prep Time: 20 minutes (+ baking time)

Instructions:

Preheat the oven to 350°F (175°C) and line a muffin tin with paper liners.

In a bowl, mix almond flour, low protein flour, and baking powder.

Add honey or maple syrup and almond milk, and stir until well combined.

Gently fold in fresh blueberries.

Divide the batter among the muffin cups and bake for 20-25 minutes or until a toothpick inserted comes out clean.

Rice Porridge with Almond Milk and Cinnamon

Ingredients:

1/2 cup cooked rice (white or brown)
1 cup unsweetened almond milk
1/2 teaspoon ground cinnamon
1 teaspoon honey or maple syrup
Prep Time: 10 minutes

Instructions:

In a saucepan, heat cooked rice and almond milk until warm.
Stir in ground cinnamon and honey or maple syrup.

Sweet Potato Hash with Spinach and Mushrooms

Ingredients:

1 medium sweet potato, peeled and diced
1 cup fresh spinach leaves
1 cup sliced mushrooms
1 tablespoon olive oil
Salt and pepper to taste
Prep Time: 15 minutes

Instructions:

In a skillet, heat olive oil over medium heat.
Add diced sweet potato and cook until tender.
Stir in spinach and mushrooms and cook until
wilted.

Banana and Almond Butter Smoothie

Ingredients:

1 ripe banana
2 tablespoons almond butter
1 cup unsweetened coconut milk
Ice cubes (optional)
Prep Time: 5 minutes

Instructions:

In a blender, combine banana, almond butter, and
coconut milk.
Blend until smooth and add ice cubes if desired.

Buckwheat Pancakes with Raspberry Sauce

Ingredients:

1 cup buckwheat flour
1 tablespoon honey or maple syrup
1 teaspoon baking powder

1 cup unsweetened almond milk

Fresh raspberries for topping

Prep Time: 15 minutes (+ cooking time)

Instructions:

In a bowl, mix buckwheat flour, honey or maple syrup, and baking powder.

Gradually add almond milk and whisk until smooth.

Heat a non-stick skillet over medium heat and pour the pancake batter.

Cook until bubbles form on the surface, then flip and cook the other side.

Top with fresh raspberries.

Polenta with Roasted Vegetables

Ingredients:

1/2 cup cooked polenta

1 cup mixed roasted vegetables (zucchini, bell peppers, eggplant)

Fresh herbs (thyme, rosemary) for topping

Prep Time: 20 minutes (+ roasting time)

Instructions:

Prepare polenta according to package instructions.

Arrange roasted vegetables over the polenta.

Garnish with fresh herbs.

Apple Cinnamon Baked Oatmeal

Ingredients:

1 cup rolled oats

1 cup unsweetened almond milk

1 apple, diced

1 teaspoon ground cinnamon

1 tablespoon honey or maple syrup

Prep Time: 10 minutes (+ baking time)

Instructions:

Preheat the oven to 375°F (190°C) and grease a baking dish.

In a bowl, mix oats, almond milk, diced apple, ground cinnamon, and honey or maple syrup.

Pour the mixture into the baking dish and spread evenly.

Bake for 25-30 minutes or until the top is golden and the oats are cooked.

Lemon Poppy Seed Muffins

Ingredients:

1 cup low protein flour (rice or oat flour)

1/4 cup honey or maple syrup

1/2 teaspoon baking powder

Zest of 1 lemon

2 tablespoons poppy seeds

1/2 cup unsweetened almond milk

Prep Time: 20 minutes (+ baking time)

Instructions:

Preheat the oven to 350°F (175°C) and line a muffin tin with paper liners.

In a bowl, mix low protein flour, honey or maple syrup, baking powder, lemon zest, and poppy seeds.

Add almond milk and stir until well combined.

Divide the batter among the muffin cups and bake for 15-20 minutes or until a toothpick inserted comes out clean.

Spinach and Feta Egg Cups

Ingredients:

4 large eggs

1 cup fresh spinach, chopped

1/4 cup crumbled feta cheese

Salt and pepper to taste

Prep Time: 15 minutes (+ baking time)

Instructions:

Preheat the oven to 375°F (190°C) and grease a muffin tin.

In a bowl, whisk eggs, chopped spinach, feta cheese, salt, and pepper.

Pour the mixture into the muffin cups, filling each about two-thirds full.

Bake for 15-20 minutes or until the egg cups are set.

Coconut Chia Pudding with Mango

Ingredients:

2 tablespoons chia seeds

1 cup coconut milk

1 tablespoon honey or maple syrup

1 ripe mango, diced

Prep Time: 5 minutes (+ 4 hours for chilling)

Instructions:

In a bowl, mix chia seeds, coconut milk, and honey or maple syrup.

Stir well and refrigerate for at least 4 hours or overnight.

Before serving, top with diced mango.

Almond Flour Waffles

Ingredients:

1 cup almond flour

1/4 cup low protein flour (rice or oat flour)

1/2 teaspoon baking powder

1 tablespoon honey or maple syrup

1 cup unsweetened almond milk

A splash of vanilla extract

Prep Time: 15 minutes (+ cooking time)

Instructions:

Preheat the waffle iron according to the manufacturer's instructions.

In a bowl, mix almond flour, low protein flour, baking powder, honey or maple syrup, almond milk, and vanilla extract.

Pour the batter onto the preheated waffle iron and cook until golden and crispy.

Pomegranate and Pistachio Yogurt Parfait

Ingredients:

1 cup low protein yogurt

1/4 cup pomegranate arils

2 tablespoons crushed pistachios

Prep Time: 5 minutes

Instructions:

In a glass or a bowl, layer low protein yogurt, pomegranate arils, and crushed pistachios.

Zucchini and Carrot Fritters

Ingredients:

1 medium zucchini, grated

1 medium carrot, grated

1/4 cup low protein flour (rice or oat flour)

1 teaspoon ground cumin

Salt and pepper to taste

Olive oil for frying

Prep Time: 20 minutes (+ frying time)

Instructions:

In a bowl, mix grated zucchini, grated carrot, low protein flour, ground cumin, salt, and pepper.

Heat olive oil in a skillet over medium heat.

Spoon the fritter mixture into the skillet and flatten with a spatula.

Cook until golden brown on both sides.

Vanilla Almond Smoothie

Ingredients:

1 cup unsweetened almond milk

1 ripe banana

1/2 teaspoon almond extract

A splash of vanilla extract

Ice cubes (optional)

Prep Time: 5 minutes

Instructions:

In a blender, combine almond milk, ripe banana, almond extract, and vanilla extract.

Blend until smooth and add ice cubes if desired.

These 20 breakfast recipes are delicious and nutritionally balanced, providing individuals with kidney disease with a diverse range of satisfying and kidney-friendly options to start their day. Remember to consult with a healthcare professional or a registered dietitian to customize the recipes according to individual dietary needs and restrictions.

Lunch Recipes

Quinoa Salad with Lemon Vinaigrette

Ingredients:

1 cup cooked quinoa

1 cup diced cucumbers

1 cup halved cherry tomatoes

1/4 cup chopped fresh parsley

Lemon vinaigrette dressing (1/4 cup olive oil, 2
tablespoons lemon juice, 1 teaspoon Dijon mustard,
salt, and pepper)

Prep Time: 15 minutes

Instructions:

In a large bowl, combine cooked quinoa, diced
cucumbers, halved cherry tomatoes, and chopped
parsley.

In a separate bowl, whisk together olive oil, lemon
juice, Dijon mustard, salt, and pepper to make the
vinaigrette.

Pour the vinaigrette over the quinoa salad and toss
to combine.

Eggplant and Tomato Stacks with Pesto

Ingredients:

1 medium eggplant, sliced

2 large tomatoes, sliced

Pesto sauce (store-bought or homemade)

Prep Time: 20 minutes (+ baking time for eggplant)

Instructions:

Preheat the oven to 400°F (200°C) and line a baking sheet with parchment paper.

Brush eggplant slices with olive oil and arrange them on the baking sheet.

Bake the eggplant slices for 15-20 minutes until tender.

Assemble the stacks by layering eggplant slices, tomato slices, and a dollop of pesto between each layer.

Lentil and Vegetable Curry

Ingredients:

1 cup cooked green lentils

1 cup chopped mixed vegetables (carrots, bell peppers, zucchini)

1 cup coconut milk

1 tablespoon curry powder

Salt and pepper to taste

Prep Time: 25 minutes

Instructions:

In a saucepan, sauté chopped vegetables until slightly softened.

Add cooked lentils, coconut milk, curry powder, salt, and pepper.

Simmer for 10-15 minutes until the vegetables are cooked and the flavors have blended.

Vegetable and Tofu Stir-Fry

Ingredients:

1 cup cubed tofu

2 cups mixed stir-fry vegetables (broccoli, bell peppers, snap peas)

2 tablespoons low sodium soy sauce

1 tablespoon sesame oil

Prep Time: 20 minutes

Instructions:

In a non-stick skillet, heat sesame oil over medium heat.

Add cubed tofu and stir-fry until lightly browned.

Add mixed vegetables and cook until tender-crisp.

Stir in low sodium soy sauce and toss to coat.

Beanless Vegetarian Chili

Ingredients:

1 cup diced tomatoes

1 cup chopped bell peppers

1 cup chopped zucchini

1 cup vegetable broth

1 teaspoon chili powder

1/2 teaspoon cumin

Salt and pepper to taste

Prep Time: 25 minutes

Instructions:

In a large pot, sauté chopped bell peppers and zucchini until softened.

Add diced tomatoes, vegetable broth, chili powder, cumin, salt, and pepper.

Simmer for 15-20 minutes until the flavors combine.

Roasted Vegetable Wrap

Ingredients:

Whole-grain tortilla

Roasted vegetables (zucchini, bell peppers, eggplant)

Low protein hummus or avocado spread

Fresh spinach leaves

Prep Time: 15 minutes (+ roasting time for vegetables)

Instructions:

Preheat the oven to 400 degrees Fahrenheit (200 degrees Celsius) and line a baking sheet with parchment paper.

Toss chopped vegetables with olive oil, salt, and pepper, and roast for 15-20 minutes.

Spread a layer of hummus or avocado spread on the tortilla.

Add roasted vegetables and fresh spinach leaves, then roll up the tortilla to make a wrap.

Cauliflower Fried Rice

Ingredients:

1 cup grated cauliflower (cauliflower rice)

1/2 cup diced carrots and peas

2 tablespoons low sodium soy sauce

1 tablespoon olive oil

Prep Time: 15 minutes

Instructions:

Warm the olive oil in a large pan over medium heat.
Add grated cauliflower and sauté for 2-3 minutes.
Stir in diced carrots and peas and cook until tender.
Drizzle low sodium soy sauce over the cauliflower rice and toss to coat.

Lentil and Rice Pilaf

Ingredients:

1/2 cup cooked green lentils

1/2 cup cooked white or brown rice

1/4 cup chopped carrots and bell peppers

1 tablespoon chopped fresh herbs (parsley, cilantro)

Lemon juice and olive oil for dressing

Prep Time: 20 minutes

Instructions:

In a bowl, combine cooked lentils, cooked rice, chopped carrots, bell peppers, and fresh herbs.

Toss with the lemon juice and olive oil to mix.

Tofu and Vegetable Lettuce Wraps

Ingredients:

Firm tofu, crumbled

Mixed diced vegetables (bell peppers, carrots, water chestnuts)

Low sodium hoisin sauce

Lettuce leaves (butter lettuce or iceberg lettuce)

Prep Time: 20 minutes

Instructions:

In a non-stick skillet, sauté crumbled tofu and diced vegetables until cooked.

Stir in low sodium hoisin sauce and toss to coat.

Spoon the tofu and vegetable mixture onto lettuce leaves and wrap to make lettuce wraps.

Baked Sweet Potato Fries

Ingredients:

2 medium sweet potatoes, cut into fries

1 tablespoon olive oil

Salt and paprika to taste

Prep Time: 15 minutes (+ baking time)

Instructions:

Preheat the oven to 220 degrees Celsius and line a baking sheet with parchment paper.

Toss sweet potato fries with olive oil, salt, and paprika.

Arrange the fries in a single layer on the baking sheet.

Bake for 20-25 minutes until crispy.

Lemon Herb Grilled Chicken (low protein portion)

Ingredients:

Low protein portion of boneless, skinless chicken breast

Lemon juice

Chopped fresh herbs (rosemary, thyme, parsley)

Olive oil

Salt and pepper to taste

Prep Time: 10 minutes (+ grilling time)

Instructions:

In a bowl, marinate the low protein portion of chicken with lemon juice, chopped fresh herbs, olive oil, salt, and pepper.

Preheat the grill to medium heat and grill the chicken until cooked through.

Zucchini Noodles with Pesto Sauce

Ingredients:

2 medium zucchini, spiralized into noodles

Pesto sauce (store-bought or homemade)

Cherry tomatoes for topping

Prep Time: 15 minutes

Instructions:

In a large skillet, sauté zucchini noodles for 2-3 minutes until tender.

Toss zucchini noodles with pesto sauce until well coated.

Top with halved cherry tomatoes.

Quinoa Stuffed Bell Peppers

Ingredients:

2 large bell peppers, halved and seeded

1 cup cooked quinoa

1 cup chopped mixed vegetables (zucchini, carrots, corn)

Low sodium vegetable broth

Salt and pepper to taste

Prep Time: 25 minutes (+ baking time)

Instructions:

Preheat the oven to 375°F (190°C) and coat a baking dish with cooking spray.

Combine cooked quinoa and chopped veggies in a mixing basin.

Fill each halved bell pepper with the quinoa and vegetable mixture.

Place the stuffed peppers in the baking dish and pour low sodium vegetable broth into the dish.

Cover with foil and bake for 25-30 minutes until the peppers are tender.

Portobello Mushroom Burgers

Ingredients:

Portobello mushroom caps

Balsamic vinegar

Olive oil

Salt and pepper to taste

Prep Time: 10 minutes (+ grilling time)

Instructions:

Preheat the grill to medium heat.

Brush portobello mushroom caps with balsamic vinegar and olive oil.

Grill the mushroom caps for 5-6 minutes on each side until tender.

Mediterranean Chickpea Salad

Ingredients:

1 can chickpeas, drained and rinsed

1 cup diced cucumbers

1 cup halved cherry tomatoes

Chopped fresh parsley and mint

Lemon juice and olive oil for dressing

Prep Time: 15 minutes

Instructions:

In a bowl, combine chickpeas, diced cucumbers, halved cherry tomatoes, chopped fresh parsley, and mint.

Toss with the lemon juice and olive oil to mix.

Spinach and Feta Stuffed Portobello Mushrooms

Ingredients:

Portobello mushroom caps

1 cup fresh spinach leaves

Crumbled feta cheese

Olive oil

Salt and pepper to taste

Prep Time: 20 minutes (+ baking time)

Instructions:

Preheat the oven to 375°F (190°C) and line a baking sheet with parchment paper.

In a non-stick skillet, sauté fresh spinach leaves until wilted.

Fill each portobello mushroom cap with sautéed spinach and crumbled feta cheese.

Season with salt and pepper and drizzle with olive oil.

Bake for 15-20 minutes until the mushrooms are tender.

Low Protein Chicken and Vegetable Stir-Fry

Ingredients:

Low protein portion of boneless, skinless chicken breast, sliced

Mixed stir-fry vegetables (broccoli, bell peppers, snap peas)

Low sodium soy sauce

Sesame oil

Prep Time: 20 minutes

Instructions:

Stir-fry sliced chicken in a nonstick pan until done.
Cook until the veggies are tender-crisp.
Toss the stir-fry with low sodium soy sauce and
sesame oil to coat.

Baked Salmon with Lemon and Dill

Ingredients:

Low protein portion of salmon fillet

Lemon juice

Fresh dill

Olive oil

Salt and pepper to taste

Prep Time: 15 minutes (+ baking time)

Instructions:

Preheat the oven to 375°F (190°C) and line a baking
sheet with parchment paper.

Place the low protein portion of salmon fillet on the
baking sheet.

Drizzle with lemon juice and olive oil, and season
with fresh dill, salt, and pepper.

Bake for 15-20 minutes until the salmon is cooked through.

Stuffed Zucchini Boats

Ingredients:

2 medium zucchini, halved and scooped

1 cup cooked quinoa or rice

1/2 cup chopped mixed vegetables (bell peppers, carrots, mushrooms)

Low sodium tomato sauce

Prep Time: 25 minutes (+ baking time)

Instructions:

Preheat the oven to 375°F (190°C) and grease a baking dish.

In a bowl, mix cooked quinoa or rice and chopped vegetables.

Fill each zucchini half with the quinoa and vegetable mixture.

Place the stuffed zucchini boats in the baking dish and pour low sodium tomato sauce over them.

Cover with foil and bake for 20-25 minutes until the zucchini is tender.

Vegetable and Tofu Noodle Soup

Ingredients:

Low protein rice noodles or shirataki noodles

Mixed diced vegetables (carrots, bell peppers, broccoli)

Cubed firm tofu

Low sodium vegetable broth

Low sodium soy sauce

Prep Time: 20 minutes

Instructions:

Bring low sodium vegetable broth to a boil in a saucepan.

Cook until the veggies and tofu are soft.

Cook until the low protein rice noodles or shirataki noodles are tender.

To taste, season with reduced sodium soy sauce.

Dinner Recipes

Baked Chicken with Herbs

Ingredients:

Low protein portion of boneless, skinless chicken breast

Chopped fresh herbs (rosemary, thyme, parsley)

Lemon juice

Olive oil

Salt and pepper to taste

Prep Time: 10 minutes (+ baking time)

Instructions:

Preheat the oven to 375°F (190°C) and line a baking sheet with parchment paper.

Place the low protein chicken breast on a baking sheet.

Season with chopped fresh herbs, salt, and pepper and drizzle with lemon juice and olive oil.

Bake for 20-25 minutes, or until the chicken is well done.

Quinoa and Vegetable Stir-Fry

Ingredients:

1 cup cooked quinoa

Mixed stir-fry vegetables (bell peppers, broccoli, snap peas)

Low-sodium soy sauce

Sesame oil

Prep Time: 20 minutes

Instructions:

Stir-fry mixed veggies in a nonstick pan until tender-crisp.

Cook until the quinoa is heated thoroughly.

Toss the stir-fry with low sodium soy sauce and sesame oil to coat.

Stuffed Bell Peppers with Lentils and Rice

Ingredients:

2 large bell peppers, halved and seeded

1 cup cooked green lentils

1 cup cooked white or brown rice

Chopped fresh parsley and cilantro

Low sodium vegetable broth

Prep Time: 30 minutes (+ baking time)

Instructions:

Preheat the oven to 190°C (375°F) and grease a baking dish.

Combine cooked lentils, cooked rice, fresh parsley, and cilantro in a mixing basin.

Fill each bell pepper half with the lentil-rice mixture.

Place the filled peppers in the baking dish and cover with low sodium vegetable broth.

Bake for 25-30 minutes, or until the peppers are cooked, covered with foil.

Lemon Herb Baked Salmon

Ingredients:

Low protein portion of salmon fillet

Lemon juice

Chopped fresh herbs (dill, parsley)

Olive oil

Salt and pepper to taste

Prep Time: 15 minutes (+ baking time)

Instructions:

Preheat the oven to 375°F (190°C) and line a baking sheet with parchment paper.

Place the low protein portion of salmon fillet on the baking sheet.

Season with lemon juice and olive oil, and season with chopped fresh herbs, salt, and pepper.

Bake for 15-20 minutes until the salmon is cooked through.

Cauliflower Rice and Vegetable Stir-Fry

Ingredients:

2 cups grated cauliflower (cauliflower rice)

Mixed stir-fry vegetables (carrots, bell peppers, snap peas)

Low sodium soy sauce

Olive oil

Prep Time: 20 minutes

Instructions:

In a large skillet, heat olive oil over medium heat.

Add grated cauliflower and stir-fry for 2-3 minutes.

Stir in mixed vegetables and cook until tender-crisp.

Add low sodium soy sauce over the stir-fry and toss to coat.

Mediterranean Chickpea Stew

Ingredients:

1 can chickpeas, drained and rinsed
1 cup diced tomatoes
1 cup chopped bell peppers
Chopped fresh parsley and oregano
Olive oil
Salt and pepper to taste

Prep Time: 25 minutes

Instructions:

In a pot, sauté chopped bell peppers in olive oil until slightly softened.
Add diced tomatoes and chickpeas, and simmer for 15-20 minutes.
Season with chopped fresh parsley, oregano, salt, and pepper.

Lemon Garlic Shrimp Skewers

Ingredients:

Low protein portion of shrimp
Lemon juice
Minced garlic

Olive oil

Fresh herbs (rosemary, thyme)

Salt and pepper to taste

Prep Time: 15 minutes (+ grilling time)

Instructions:

Heat the grill to medium-high.

Marinate the shrimp with lemon juice, chopped garlic, olive oil, fresh herbs, salt, and pepper in a basin.

Thread the shrimp onto skewers and grill for 2-3 minutes each side, or until done.

Baked Eggplant Parmesan

Ingredients:

1 medium eggplant, sliced

Low sodium marinara sauce

Low protein mozzarella cheese

Fresh basil leaves

Prep Time: 30 minutes (+ baking time)

Instructions:

Preheat the oven to 375°F (190°C) and line a baking sheet with parchment paper.

Arrange the eggplant slices on the baking pan and brush with olive oil.

Bake for 15-20 minutes, or until the eggplant slices are soft.

Layer eggplant slices, low sodium marinara sauce, low protein mozzarella cheese, and fresh basil leaves in a baking dish.

Bake until the cheese is melted and bubbling, then repeat the layers.

Zucchini Noodles with Avocado Pesto

Ingredients:

2 medium zucchini, spiralized into noodles
Avocado pesto sauce (1 ripe avocado, basil leaves, garlic, lemon juice, olive oil, salt, and pepper)

Prep Time: 20 minutes

Instructions:

To create the avocado pesto sauce, combine ripe avocado, basil leaves, garlic, lemon juice, olive oil, salt, and pepper in a food processor.

Sauté zucchini noodles in a large pan for 2-3 minutes, or until soft.
Toss zucchini noodles in avocado pesto sauce until well covered.

Tofu and Vegetable Stir-Fry

Ingredients:

Cubed firm tofu
Mixed stir-fry vegetables (bell peppers, broccoli, snap peas)
Low sodium soy sauce
Sesame oil

Prep Time: 20 minutes

Instructions:

Stir-fry cubed tofu in a nonstick pan until lightly browned.
Cook until the veggies are tender-crisp.
Toss the stir-fry with low sodium soy sauce and sesame oil to coat.

Butternut Squash and Sage Risotto

Ingredients:

1 cup cooked butternut squash, mashed

1 cup Arborio rice

Chopped fresh sage leaves

Low sodium vegetable broth

Olive oil

Salt and pepper to taste

Prep Time: 30 minutes

Instructions:

In a large saucepan, sauté Arborio rice in olive oil until lightly toasted.

Gradually add low sodium vegetable broth, stirring continuously, until the rice is cooked and creamy.

Stir in mashed butternut squash and chopped fresh sage leaves.

Season with salt and pepper

Stuffed Portobello Mushrooms with Spinach and Feta

Ingredients:

Portobello mushroom caps

Fresh spinach leaves

Crumbled feta cheese

Olive oil

Salt and pepper to taste

Prep Time: 25 minutes (+ baking time)

Instructions:

Preheat the oven to 375°F (190°C) and line a baking sheet with parchment paper.

Sauté fresh spinach leaves on a nonstick pan until wilted.

Fill each portobello mushroom cap with sautéed spinach and feta cheese crumbles.

Season with salt and pepper and drizzle with olive oil.

Bake the mushrooms for 15-20 minutes, or until they are soft.

Cilantro Lime Shrimp with Cauliflower Rice

Ingredients:

Low protein portion of shrimp

Chopped fresh cilantro

Lime juice

Grated cauliflower (cauliflower rice)

Olive oil

Salt and pepper to taste

Prep Time: 20 minutes

Instructions:

Marinate the shrimp with chopped fresh cilantro,
lime juice, olive oil, salt, and pepper in a bowl.
Sauté grated cauliflower in a large pan until soft.
Cook the marinated shrimp in a separate pan until
pink and opaque.

Tomato Basil Spaghetti Squash

Ingredients:

1 medium spaghetti squash, cooked and shredded
Low sodium marinara sauce
Fresh basil leaves
Olive oil
Salt and pepper to taste

Prep Time: 30 minutes (+ cooking time for
spaghetti squash)

Instructions:

Preheat the oven to 375°F (190°C).

Remove the seeds from the spaghetti squash and cut it in half lengthwise.

On a baking sheet, sprinkle the squash halves with olive oil and season with salt and pepper.

30-40 minutes, or until the squash is soft.

Shred the cooked spaghetti squash with a fork to make "noodles."

Heat low sodium marinara sauce in a pot.

Toss the warm marinara sauce with the shredded spaghetti squash.

Garnish with fresh basil leaves if desired.

Ratatouille

Ingredients:

1 cup diced tomatoes

1 cup diced eggplant

1 cup diced zucchini

1 cup diced bell peppers

Chopped fresh basil and thyme

Olive oil

Salt and pepper to taste

Prep Time: 30 minutes

Instructions:

Sauté chopped eggplant in olive oil in a large pan until tender.

Cook until the zucchini and bell peppers are soft.

Cook until all of the veggies are soft, about 10 minutes.

Season with fresh basil, thyme, salt, and pepper to taste.

Low Protein Portion Beef and Broccoli Stir-Fry

Ingredients:

Low protein portion of beef, sliced

Broccoli florets

Low sodium soy sauce

Olive oil

Prep Time: 20 minutes

Instructions:

Stir-fry sliced beef in a skillet until cooked.

Add broccoli florets and cook until it is tender-crisp.

Sprinkle low sodium soy sauce over the stir-fry and toss to coat.

Lemon Herb Grilled Chicken with Quinoa

Ingredients:

Low protein portion of boneless, skinless chicken breast

Lemon juice

Chopped fresh herbs (rosemary, thyme, parsley)

Olive oil

Salt and pepper to taste

1 cup cooked quinoa

Prep Time: 15 minutes (+ grilling time)

Instructions:

Preheat the grill to medium heat.

Marinate the low protein portion of chicken breast with lemon juice, chopped fresh herbs, olive oil, salt, and pepper in a bowl.

Grill the chicken until well cooked.

Serve the grilled chicken over cooked quinoa.

Low Protein Portion Beef and Vegetable Stir-Fry

Ingredients:

Low protein portion of beef, sliced
Stir-fry mixed vegetables (bell peppers, broccoli,
snap peas)
Low sodium soy sauce
Olive oil

Prep Time: 20 minutes

Instructions:

In a non-stick skillet, stir-fry sliced beef until
cooked.
Add mixed vegetables and cook until tender-crisp.
Drizzle low sodium soy sauce over the stir-fry and
toss to coat.

Low Protein Portion Chicken and Vegetable Skewers

Ingredients:

Low protein portion of boneless, skinless chicken
breast, cubed
Mixed diced vegetables (bell peppers, zucchini,
onions)
Olive oil
Fresh herbs (thyme, rosemary)
Salt and pepper to taste

Prep Time: 15 minutes (+ grilling time)

Instructions:

Heat the grill to medium-high.

Thread skewers with cubed chicken and diced veggies.

Drizzle with olive oil and season with salt and pepper.

Grill the skewers for 2-3 minutes each side, or until the chicken is thoroughly cooked.

Stuffed Mushrooms with Spinach and Feta

Ingredients:

Large mushroom caps

Fresh spinach leaves

Crumbled feta cheese

Olive oil

Salt and pepper to taste

Prep Time: 20 minutes (+ baking time)

Instructions:

Preheat the oven to 190 degrees Celsius and line a baking sheet with parchment paper.

Sauté fresh spinach leaves on a nonstick pan until wilted.

Fill each mushroom cap with sautéed spinach and feta cheese crumbles.

Season with salt and pepper and drizzle with olive oil.

Bake the mushrooms for 15-20 minutes, or until they are soft.

Soup and Stew Recipes

Vegetable and Lentil Soup

Ingredients:

1 cup cooked green lentils

Mixed chopped vegetables (carrots, celery, onions)

Low sodium vegetable broth

Chopped fresh herbs (parsley, thyme)

Olive oil

Salt and pepper to taste

Prep Time: 25 minutes

Instructions:

Sauté chopped onions, carrots, and celery in olive oil until softened in a saucepan.

Bring cooked lentils and reduced sodium vegetable broth to a boil.

Cook the veggies until they are soft.

Season with fresh herbs, salt, and pepper to taste.

Tomato Basil Soup

Ingredients:

1 cup diced tomatoes

Chopped fresh basil

Low sodium vegetable broth

Olive oil

Salt and pepper to taste

Prep Time: 20 minutes

Instructions:

Cook chopped tomatoes in olive oil until softened in a saucepan.

Bring to a simmer with reduced sodium vegetable broth.

Cook for around 15 minutes.

Using a blender or immersion blender, puree the soup.

Add the fresh basil, salt, and pepper to taste.

Butternut Squash Soup

Ingredients:

1 cup cooked butternut squash, mashed

Low sodium vegetable broth

Chopped fresh thyme

Olive oil

Salt and pepper to taste

Prep Time: 30 minutes

Instructions:

Sauté mashed butternut squash in olive oil in a saucepan until warmed.

Bring to a simmer with reduced sodium vegetable broth.

Cook for 15-20 minutes, or until the flavors combine.

Season with freshly chopped thyme, salt, and pepper.

Spinach and Potato Soup

Ingredients:

2 cups fresh spinach leaves

1 cup diced potatoes

Low sodium vegetable broth

Chopped fresh dill

Olive oil

Salt and pepper to taste

Prep Time: 25 minutes

Instructions:

Sauté chopped potatoes in olive oil in a saucepan until slightly softened.

Bring to a simmer with reduced sodium vegetable broth.

Cook the potatoes until they are soft.

Cook until fresh spinach leaves are wilted.

Season with freshly chopped dill, salt, and pepper.

Carrot Ginger Soup

Ingredients:

2 cups chopped carrots

Fresh ginger, grated

Low sodium vegetable broth

Coconut milk

Olive oil

Salt and pepper to taste

Prep Time: 25 minutes

Instructions:

In a saucepan, heat olive oil and sauté chopped carrots and grated ginger until slightly softened.

Bring to a simmer with reduced sodium vegetable broth.

Cook the carrots until they are soft.

Using a blender or immersion blender, puree the soup.

Season with salt and pepper after adding the coconut milk.

Soup with chicken and rice (poor in protein)

Chicken and Rice Soup (low protein portion)

Ingredients:

Low protein portion of boneless, skinless chicken breast, diced

Cooked white or brown rice

Mixed chopped vegetables (carrots, celery, onions)

Low sodium chicken broth

Chopped fresh parsley

Olive oil

Salt and pepper to taste

Prep Time: 30 minutes

Instructions:

In a pot, sauté diced chicken in olive oil until cooked.

Add mixed vegetables and cook until softened.

Add low sodium chicken broth and bring to a simmer.

Stir in cooked rice and cook until heated through.

Season with chopped fresh parsley, salt, and pepper.

Sweet Potato and Black Bean Chili

Ingredients:

1 cup diced sweet potatoes

1 can black beans, drained and rinsed

Chopped bell peppers

Diced tomatoes

Chili powder

Low sodium vegetable broth

Olive oil

Salt and pepper to taste

Prep Time: 30 minutes

Instructions:

In a pot, sauté diced sweet potatoes and chopped bell peppers in olive oil until slightly softened.

Add diced tomatoes, black beans, and chili powder.

Pour in low sodium vegetable broth and bring to a simmer.

Cook until the sweet potatoes are tender.

Season with salt and pepper.

Low Protein Portion Beef and Vegetable Stew

Ingredients:

Low protein portion of beef, cubed

Mixed chopped vegetables (carrots, potatoes, onions)

Low sodium beef broth

Chopped fresh thyme and rosemary

Olive oil

Salt and pepper to taste

Prep Time: 30 minutes

Instructions:

Sear cubed beef in olive oil in a skillet until browned.

Cook until the veggies are somewhat softened.

Bring to a simmer with reduced sodium beef broth.

Cook the meat until it is tender.

Season with fresh thyme, rosemary, salt, and pepper to taste.

Egg Drop Soup

Ingredients:

Low sodium chicken broth

Eggs, beaten

Sliced green onions

Fresh ginger, grated

Low sodium soy sauce

Sesame oil

Prep Time: 15 minutes

Instructions:

Bring low sodium chicken broth to a boil in a saucepan.

To make ribbons of cooked egg, slowly trickle beaten eggs into the boiling soup while gently swirling.

Stir in the cut green onions and fresh ginger.

Season with sesame oil and low sodium soy sauce.

Vegetable and Barley Soup

Ingredients:

Cooked barley

Mixed chopped vegetables (carrots, celery, zucchini)

Low sodium vegetable broth

Chopped fresh thyme and parsley

Olive oil

Salt and pepper to taste

Prep Time: 25 minutes

Instructions:

Sauté chopped carrots, celery, and zucchini in olive oil in a saucepan until slightly softened.

Bring to a simmer with reduced sodium vegetable broth.

Cook until the cooked barley is heated thoroughly.

Season with fresh thyme, parsley, salt, and pepper to taste.

Minestrone Soup

Ingredients:

Cooked low protein pasta (such as rice or corn pasta)

Mixed chopped vegetables (carrots, celery, zucchini)

Low sodium vegetable broth

Diced tomatoes

Cooked white beans

Chopped fresh basil and oregano

Olive oil

Salt and pepper to taste

Prep Time: 30 minutes

Instructions:

Sauté chopped carrots, celery, and zucchini in olive oil in a saucepan until slightly softened.

Cooked white beans, sliced tomatoes, and low sodium vegetable broth are all good additions.

Cook until the veggies are soft, about 20 minutes.

Mix in the cooked low-protein pasta.

Season with fresh basil, oregano, salt, and pepper to taste.

Miso Soup with Tofu and Seaweed

Ingredients:

Low sodium miso paste

Cubed firm tofu

Wakame seaweed, soaked and chopped

Sliced green onions

Low sodium vegetable broth

Prep Time: 15 minutes

Instructions:

Bring low sodium vegetable broth to a boil in a saucepan.

Miso paste, dissolved in a tiny amount of warm water, is added to the boiling soup.

Toss in the cubed tofu and chopped wakame seaweed.

Cook for a few minutes, or until the seaweed wilts.

Garnish with green onions, sliced.

Low Protein Portion Chicken and Vegetable Soup

Ingredients:

Low protein portion of boneless, skinless chicken breast, diced

Mixed chopped vegetables (carrots, celery, onions)

Low sodium chicken broth

Cooked white or brown rice

Chopped fresh parsley

Olive oil

Salt and pepper to taste

Prep Time: 30 minutes

Instructions:

In a pot, sauté diced chicken in olive oil until cooked.

Cook until the mixed veggies are softened.

Bring to a simmer with reduced sodium chicken broth.

Cook until the cooked rice is heated thoroughly.

Season with freshly chopped parsley, salt, and pepper.

Roasted Red Pepper and Tomato Soup

Ingredients:

Roasted red peppers, diced

Diced tomatoes

Chopped onions

Low sodium vegetable broth

Fresh basil leaves

Olive oil

Salt and pepper to taste

Prep Time: 30 minutes

Instructions:

In a saucepan, sauté chopped onions in olive oil until softened.

Toss in the roasted red peppers and chopped tomatoes.

Bring to a simmer with reduced sodium vegetable broth.

Cook for around 15 minutes.

Using a blender or immersion blender, puree the soup.

Add the chopped fresh basil leaves, salt, and pepper to taste.

Potato Leek Soup

Ingredients:

Chopped leeks

Diced potatoes

Low sodium vegetable broth

Low sodium soy milk or almond milk

Olive oil

Salt and pepper to taste

Prep Time: 25 minutes

Instructions:

In a saucepan, sauté chopped leeks in olive oil until softened.

Combine chopped potatoes and low sodium vegetable broth in a mixing bowl.

Cook until the potatoes are soft, about 20 minutes.

Using a blender or immersion blender, puree the soup.

Add low sodium soy milk or almond milk, salt, and pepper to taste.

Black-Eyed Pea and Vegetable Stew

Ingredients:

Cooked black-eyed peas

Mixed chopped vegetables (carrots, bell peppers, onions)

Low sodium vegetable broth

Chopped fresh thyme and parsley

Olive oil

Salt and pepper to taste

Prep Time: 25 minutes

Instructions:

Sauté chopped onions, carrots, and bell peppers in olive oil in a saucepan until slightly softened.
Bring to a simmer with reduced sodium vegetable broth.
Cook until the black-eyed peas are heated through.
Season with fresh thyme, parsley, salt, and pepper to taste.

Cauliflower and Broccoli Soup

Ingredients:

2 cups chopped cauliflower

2 cups chopped broccoli

Low sodium vegetable broth

Low sodium soy milk or almond milk

Chopped fresh thyme and rosemary

Olive oil

Salt and pepper to taste

Prep Time: 30 minutes

Instructions:

Sauté chopped cauliflower and broccoli in olive oil in a saucepan until slightly softened.

Bring to a simmer with reduced sodium vegetable broth.

Cook the veggies until they are soft.

Using a blender or immersion blender, puree the soup.

Add low sodium soy milk or almond milk, fresh thyme, rosemary, salt, and pepper to taste.

Lentil and Vegetable Stew

Ingredients:

1 cup cooked green lentils

Mixed chopped vegetables (carrots, celery, bell peppers)

Low sodium vegetable broth

Chopped fresh thyme and parsley

Olive oil

Salt and pepper to taste

Prep Time: 25 minutes

Instructions:

Sauté chopped carrots, celery, and bell peppers in olive oil in a saucepan until slightly softened.

Bring to a simmer with reduced sodium vegetable broth.

Cook until the cooked green lentils are heated thoroughly.

Season with fresh thyme, parsley, salt, and pepper to taste.

Spicy Red Lentil Soup

Ingredients:

1 cup red lentils

Chopped onions

Diced tomatoes

Low sodium vegetable broth

Ground cumin

Ground coriander

Olive oil

Salt and pepper to taste

Prep Time: 25 minutes

Instructions:

In a saucepan, sauté chopped onions in olive oil until softened.

Cook for a few minutes after adding the diced tomatoes.

Bring to a simmer with reduced sodium vegetable broth.

Stir in the red lentils, cumin, and coriander.

Cook the lentils until they are soft.

Season with salt and pepper to taste.

Cabbage and White Bean Soup

Ingredients:

Shredded cabbage

Cooked white beans

Chopped onions

Low sodium vegetable broth

Chopped fresh thyme and parsley

Olive oil

Salt and pepper to taste

Prep Time: 25 minutes

Instructions:

Sauté chopped onions in olive oil in a saucepan until tender.

Cook until the cabbage is somewhat tender.

Bring to a simmer with reduced sodium vegetable broth.

Cook until the cooked white beans are heated thoroughly.

Season with fresh thyme, parsley, salt, and pepper to taste.

Conclusion

This book is a comprehensive and useful resource for anybody coping with renal health concerns. Throughout this book, we have discussed the vital importance of a low protein diet in the management of renal illness, providing practical insights and powerful advice for readers to take ownership of their health.

At the heart of this book is the range of excellent and kidney-friendly foods featured for each mealtime. These meals show that a low protein diet can be satisfying and enjoyable, with everything from hearty breakfasts to filling lunches and hearty nights. Readers are given the skills they need to enjoy a diverse range of meals and culinary experiences, ensuring that their nutritional route is both healthy and enjoyable.

Furthermore, "Low Protein Diet for Kidney Disease" fosters a sense of community and support, stressing that persons suffering from kidney disease are not alone in their pursuit of improved health. Thanks to the advice of healthcare specialists and the companionship of others dealing with similar challenges, readers discover serenity and support as they embrace their nutritious lifestyle.

Readers go on a life-changing journey toward renal health by putting the ideals of a low protein diet into practice. Every conscious meal choice becomes an important step toward fueling their bodies, controlling their condition, and building a sense of empowerment. The book instills the idea that, with patience and commitment, kidney disease may be changed into a chance for positive development and new well-being.

Finally, "Low Protein Diet for Kidney Disease" is a beacon of light, offering a path to better health and a brighter future. By adopting the concepts of a low protein diet and making conscious lifestyle choices, readers embark on a journey of self-care and well-being. This book serves as a continuous companion, enabling people to take care of their health and equipping them with the tools they need to live life to the fullest despite the challenges of renal illness.

"Dear Readers,

As you come to the end of this journey through 'Low Protein Diet for Kidney Disease,' we extend our heartfelt gratitude for accompanying us on this path to better health. Your dedication to understanding the nuances of managing kidney disease through a low protein diet is both admirable and inspiring.

We sincerely hope that this book has provided you with the knowledge, insights, and tools you need to make informed choices about your dietary lifestyle. Your commitment to embracing a kidney-friendly approach to nutrition is a testament to your strength and determination to improve your well-being.

Remember, your health journey is unique, and every step you take towards a low protein diet is a step towards greater vitality and resilience. The information and recipes shared within these pages are meant to serve as a foundation upon which you can build your own path to kidney health.

As you navigate the challenges and triumphs of managing kidney disease, know that you are not alone. There is a community of individuals who share your journey and a network of healthcare professionals ready to support you every step of the way.

Thank you for entrusting us with a part of your wellness journey. We wish you continued success, strength, and improved health. May your commitment to a low protein diet be a beacon of hope and a source of empowerment, guiding you towards a brighter and healthier future.

30 Day Meal Plan

Day 1:

- Breakfast: Creamy oatmeal with sliced bananas and a sprinkle of cinnamon.
- Lunch: Mixed green salad with cherry tomatoes, cucumbers, and a lemon vinaigrette dressing.
- Dinner: Baked salmon with steamed asparagus and quinoa.

Day 2:

- Breakfast: Scrambled eggs with sautéed spinach and cherry tomatoes.
- Lunch: Lentil and vegetable soup with a side of whole-grain bread.
- Dinner: Grilled chicken breast with roasted sweet potatoes and green beans.

Day 3:

- Breakfast: Smoothie made with almond milk, mixed berries, and a banana.
- Lunch: Cabbage and white bean stew with a side of brown rice.
- Dinner: Stir-fried tofu with broccoli, bell peppers, and low sodium soy sauce.

Day 4:

- Breakfast: Greek yogurt with sliced peaches and a drizzle of honey.
- Lunch: Tomato basil soup with a side of whole-grain crackers.
- Dinner: Low protein portion beef and vegetable stir-fry with cauliflower rice.

Day 5:

- Breakfast: Quinoa breakfast bowl with chopped apples, almonds, and a sprinkle of nutmeg.
- Lunch: Egg drop soup with sliced green onions and grated fresh ginger.
- Dinner: Baked chicken thighs with a side of mixed steamed vegetables.

Day 6:

- Breakfast: Chia seed pudding with coconut milk and fresh berries.
- Lunch: Vegetable and barley soup with a side of whole-grain bread.
- Dinner: Roasted red pepper and tomato soup with a spinach salad.

Day 7:

- Breakfast: Avocado toast on whole-grain bread with cherry tomatoes.
- Lunch: Butternut squash soup with a side of quinoa.

- Dinner: Grilled shrimp skewers with a mixed green salad.

Day 8:

- Breakfast: Smoothie made with soy milk, mango, and a sprinkle of turmeric.
- Lunch: Miso soup with tofu and seaweed.
- Dinner: Low protein portion chicken and vegetable stir-fry with brown rice.

Day 9:

- Breakfast: Low protein portion ham and cheese omelet with spinach.
- Lunch: Cauliflower and broccoli soup with a side of whole-grain crackers.
- Dinner: Baked cod with lemon and dill, served with steamed carrots.

Day 10:

- Breakfast: Apple cinnamon pancakes made with rice flour.
- Lunch: Spinach and potato soup with a side of whole-grain bread.
- Dinner: Stuffed bell peppers with quinoa and black beans.

Day 11:

- Breakfast: Smoothie made with almond milk, pineapple, and kale.

- Lunch: Low protein portion beef and vegetable stew with a side of couscous.
- Dinner: Baked turkey breast with roasted Brussels sprouts.

Day 12:

- Breakfast: Overnight chia oats with almond milk and mixed berries.
- Lunch: Minestrone soup with a side of whole-grain bread.
- Dinner: Grilled lamb chops with a side of sautéed spinach.

Day 13:

- Breakfast: Greek yogurt parfait with honey and granola.
- Lunch: Eggplant and lentil curry with a side of brown rice.
- Dinner: Baked tilapia with lemon and herbs, served with steamed asparagus.

Day 14:

- Breakfast: Banana walnut muffins made with low protein flour.
- Lunch: Carrot ginger soup with a side of whole-grain crackers.
- Dinner: Low protein portion chicken and vegetable kebabs with a mixed green salad.

Day 15:

- Breakfast: Smoothie made with soy milk, blueberries, and spinach.
- Lunch: Black-eyed pea and vegetable stew with a side of quinoa.
- Dinner: Baked pork chops with a side of roasted sweet potatoes.

Day 16:

- Breakfast: Breakfast burrito with scrambled eggs, sautéed vegetables, and salsa.
- Lunch: Tomato basil soup with a side of whole-grain bread.
- Dinner: Grilled shrimp with a mixed green salad.

Day 17:

- Breakfast: Chia seed pudding with coconut milk and sliced peaches.
- Lunch: Lentil and vegetable soup with a side of brown rice.
- Dinner: Stir-fried tofu with broccoli, bell peppers, and low sodium soy sauce.

Day 18:

- Breakfast: Smoothie made with almond milk, strawberries, and kale.
- Lunch: Cabbage and white bean stew with a side of quinoa.
- Dinner: Low protein portion beef and vegetable stir-fry with cauliflower rice.

Day 19:

- Breakfast: Greek yogurt with honey, sliced bananas, and chopped walnuts.
- Lunch: Egg drop soup with sliced green onions and grated fresh ginger.
- Dinner: Baked chicken thighs with a side of mixed steamed vegetables.

Day 20:

- Breakfast: Quinoa breakfast bowl with mixed berries and a sprinkle of cinnamon.
- Lunch: Vegetable and barley soup with a side of whole-grain bread.
- Dinner: Roasted red pepper and tomato soup with a spinach salad.

Day 21:

- Breakfast: Smoothie made with soy milk, mixed berries, and a sprinkle of turmeric.
- Lunch: Miso soup with tofu and seaweed.
- Dinner: Low protein portion chicken and vegetable stir-fry with brown rice.

Day 22:

- Breakfast: Low protein portion ham and cheese omelet with spinach.

- Lunch: Cauliflower and broccoli soup with a side of whole-grain crackers.
- Dinner: Baked cod with lemon and dill, served with steamed carrots.

Day 23:

- Breakfast: Apple cinnamon pancakes made with rice flour.
- Lunch: Spinach and potato soup with a side of whole-grain bread.
- Dinner: Stuffed bell peppers with quinoa and black beans.

Day 24:

- Breakfast: Smoothie made with almond milk, pineapple, and kale.
- Lunch: Low protein portion beef and vegetable stew with a side of couscous.
- Dinner: Baked turkey breast with roasted Brussels sprouts.

Day 25:

- Breakfast: Overnight chia oats with almond milk and mixed berries.
- Lunch: Minestrone soup with a side of whole-grain bread.
- Dinner: Grilled lamb chops with a side of sautéed spinach.

Day 26:

- Breakfast: Greek yogurt parfait with honey and granola.
- Lunch: Eggplant and lentil curry with a side of brown rice.
- Dinner: Baked tilapia with lemon and herbs, served with steamed asparagus.

Day 27:

- Breakfast: Banana walnut muffins made with low protein flour.
- Lunch: Carrot ginger soup with a side of whole-grain crackers.
- Dinner: Low protein portion chicken and vegetable kebabs with a mixed green salad.

Day 28:

- Breakfast: Smoothie made with soy milk, blueberries, and spinach.
- Lunch: Black-eyed pea and vegetable stew with a side of quinoa.
- Dinner: Baked pork chops with a side of roasted sweet potatoes.

Day 29:

- Breakfast: Smoothie made with almond milk, mixed berries, and a sprinkle of cinnamon.
- Lunch: Lentil and vegetable soup with a side of whole-grain bread.

- Dinner: Baked salmon with steamed asparagus and quinoa.

Day 30:

- Breakfast: Scrambled eggs with sautéed spinach and cherry tomatoes.
- Lunch: Cabbage and white bean stew with a side of brown rice.
- Dinner: Grilled chicken breast with roasted sweet potatoes and green beans.

Made in United States
Orlando, FL
22 January 2024